Table of Contents

Appendicitis happens when your appendix becomes inflamed, likely due to a blockage. It can be acute or chronic.

In the United States, appendicitis is the most commonTrusted Source cause of abdominal pain resulting in surgery. Up to 9 percent of Americans experience it at some point in their lives.

The appendix is a small pouch attached to the intestine. It's located in your lower-right abdomen. When your appendix becomes blocked, bacteria can multiply inside it. This can lead to the formation of pus and swelling, which can cause painful pressure in your abdomen. Appendicitis can also block blood flow.

Left untreated, appendicitis can cause your appendix to burst. This can cause bacteria to spill into your abdominal cavity, which can be serious and sometimes fatal.

BREAKFAST

1. Avocado Breakfast Burrito.

Prep Time: 10 Minutes

Cook Time: 20 Minutes

Servings 4

Ingredients

- 4-6 slices thick cut bacon chopped
- 1 tablespoons olive oil
- 1/2 sweet onion chopped
- 1 red bell pepper chopped
- 1 poblano pepper chopped or sliced
- 1/2 cup yellow corn
- 1 clove garlic, minced or grated
- salt + pepper
- 8 eggs
- 1 1/2 cups shredded sharp cheddar cheese
- 1/4 cup fresh basil + cilantro chopped
- 1 cup leftover french fries or roasted potatoes

- 1 avocado sliced
- 4 Old El Paso Burrito Tortillas warmed

Instructions

1. Heat a large skillet or wok over medium heat. Add the bacon and cook until crisp. Drain the bacon onto a paper towel lined plate. Pour off all but 1 tablespoon of bacon grease from the skillet. Add the remaining tablespoon of grease back to the skillet, along with a small drizzle of olive oil, set the skillet back on the stove over medium heat. Add the onions, red pepper, poblano pepper and corn. Cook 5 minutes or until softened. Add the garlic and cook 30 seconds longer. Season with salt + pepper and remove from the skillet to a plate.

2. Return the skillet to medium heat and again add a drizzle of oil. Whisk together the eggs and cheese in a bowl. Pour the eggs into the skillet, scrambling until cooked through, about 3-5 minutes. Season with salt + pepper and remove from the heat. Stir in the basil + cilantro.

3. Place one tortilla at a time in the microwave for 30 seconds. Working quickly, layer the scrambled eggs,

veggies, bacon, french fries and avocado towards one end of the tortilla. Fold the tortilla over the ingredients. Roll up the tortilla (try and roll them tight). Repeat with remaining tortillas and ingredients. Roll the finished burritos in tin foil to keep them packed tight. To reheat, place the burritos in the oven for 10 minutes or until warmed through. Serve as desired with sour cream, salsa and hot sauce.

Prep Time: 10 Minutes

Cook Time: 25 Minutes

Servings 4

Ingredients

- Blueberry Muffin Granola:
- 3 cups rolled oats use gluten free if needed
- 1/2 cup raw almond roughly chopped
- 1/2 cup raw pepitas
- 1/3 cup coconut oil melted
- 1/3 cup maple syrup or honey
- 1 teaspoon vanilla
- 2 very ripe banana finely mashed
- zest of 1 lemon
- 1-2 cups fresh blueberries

For The Greek Yogurt Bowls:

- plain Greek yogurt
- fresh fruit (I like fresh berries bananas, passion fruit, pineapple + mango)
- sliced avocado optional

- nuts + seeds (I like hemp seeds chia seeds, bee pollen, almonds + pistachios)
- honey or maple for drizzling
- edible flowers optional

Instructions

1. Preheat the oven to 350 degrees F. Line a large baking sheet with parchment paper.
2. To the baking sheet, add the oats, almond and pepitas. In a small sauce pan melt together the coconut oil and maple (or honey). Once melted stir in the vanilla, mashed banana and lemon zest. Remove from the heat and pour the mixture over the oat mix, toss well and sprinkle with salt. Stir in the blueberries.
3. Bake for 25-30 minutes, stirring 1 to 2 times throughout cooking. The granola is done when the oats smell toasted and are golden brown. Allow the granola to cool completely. Store in an airtight container for up to one week.

For The Bowls

1. Spoon a little yogurt into a bowl. Top with granola, fresh fruit, avocado, seeds + nuts. Drizzle with honey

or maple and garnish with edible flowers if desired. EAT.

Prep Time: 40 Minutes

Cook Time: 20 Minutes

Servings 8

Ingredients

- 1 tablespoon olive oil
- 1 sweet onion diced
- 2 cloves garlic minced or grated
- pinch of salt and pepper
- 1 jalapeno seeded and diced
- 1 potato chopped
- 1 pound ground chorizo or chorizo with the casings removed
- 1 teaspoon cumin
- 1 teaspoon dried oregano
- 8 large eggs beaten
- 1/4 cup milk I use 2%
- 8 large flour tortillas
- canola oil if you are frying the chimichangas

Beans:

- 2 cups black beans drained and rinsed if using canned
- 1/2 teaspoon chili powder
- 1/2 teaspoon garlic powder
- salt and pepper to taste

Cilantro Avocado Crema:

- 1 cup cilantro chopped
- 2 large ripe avocdos
- 1 cup greek yogurt
- 1/2 lime juiced
- salt and pepper taste

Toppings:

- 1 cup sharp cheddar cheese shredde
- 1 cup pepper jack cheese shredded
- 1 pint grape tomatoes halved
- 1/2 cup cotija cheese crumbled
- 8-12 pickled jalapenos

Instructions

2. To make the beans. Mash the black beens until smooth, but still a little chunky. Stir in the chili, garlic powder, salt and pepper. Set aside.

3. To make the cilantro-avocado crema. In a blender or food processor, combine the cilantro, avocados, greek yogurt, lime juice and a pinch of salt + pepper. Blend until smooth. Set aside.

4. Heat a large skillet over medium heat, add 1 tablespoon olive oil. Throw in the onion and cook, stirring to coat. Cook until the onions are soft and fragrant. Add the garlic, diced jalapeños and diced potatoes. Cover and cook cook another 10 minutes. Add the chorizo, cumin and oregano. Cook, stirring until just beginning to brown, about 5 minutes. Scoop the chorizo out of the skillet with a slotted spoon and transfer to a plate. Wipe the skillet out with a paper towel.

5. Return the skillet to medium to medium-low heat and heat the remaining 1 tablespoon oil. Add the egg mixture and cook, stirring, about 3 minutes. Add the chorizo and cook, stirring about 2 to 4 minutes more depending on the desired firmness of the eggs.

6. To assemble. Warm the tortillas in a microwave for just a few seconds. Using a rubber spatula or the back of a spoon, spread a little of the beans towards the end of each tortilla. Add the chorizo + egg mixture directly over the beans. Fold the sides of the line of

ingredients and roll up the tortilla (try and roll them tight). Using some kitchen twine (or I just used some christmas string lying around), tie the twine tightly around the burrito. Repeat with the remaining ingredients.

7. To fry the chimichangas. Preheat the oven to 450 degrees. Fill a large pot with an inch of oil and bring it to 350 degrees F. When the oil is hot, add 2 burritos at a time, seam-side down, adjusting the temperature to keep the oil at 350 degrees F. Cook until golden on the bottom, then roll and cook all sides, about 3 to 5 minutes total. Transfer to a paper towel-lined plate. Repeat with the remaining chimichangas.

8. Place the chimichangas on a baking sheet and cut off the twine. Top each one with equal amounts of cheddar and pepper jack. Cook until the cheese melts, about 2-5 minutes. Transfer each to a serving plate and top evenly with cilantro-avocado crema, tomatoes, pickled jalapeños and crumbled cotija cheese.

9. To bake the chimichangas. Preheat the oven to 450 degrees F. Put the chimichangas seam-side down on the baking sheet. Bake for 4-5 minutes until crisp. Remove from the oven and top each one with equal

amounts to cheddar and pepper jack. Place back in the oven until the cheese melts, about 2-5 minutes. Transfer each to a serving plate and top evenly with cilantro-avocado crema, tomatoes, pickled jalapeños and crumbled cotija cheese.

Prep Time: 15 Minutes

Cook Time: 25 Minutes

Servings 6

Ingredients

- 6 slices thick cut bacon chopped
- 2 tablespoons olive oil
- 2 cloves garlic minced or grated
- 8 ounces cremini mushrooms sliced
- 1 teaspoon dried dill
- 1/2 teaspoon dried oregano
- 1/2 teaspoon crushed red pepper
- 1/2 teaspoon pepper
- 1/4 teaspoon salt
- 16 ounces frozen chopped spinach thawed
- 12 ounces marinated artichokes hearts drained
- 1 pound angle hair pasta
- 8 ounces fontina cheese half diced, half shredded (or more!)
- 6-8 eggs
- 2-3 tablespoons heavy cream

- lots of chopped parsley for garnish

Instructions

1. Bring a large pot of salted water to a boil. Add the pasta and prepare according to directions. Drain and set aside. Preheat the oven to 374 degrees F.

2. Heat a large skillet (mine was 12 inches) over medium-high heat and cook bacon until crispy. Remove to a paper towel-lined plate. Remove all but one tablespoon of bacon fat from the pan, then add the olive oil and heat over high heat. Add garlic and saute for 30 seconds. Add the mushrooms in a single layer. Don't stir them! Let them sizzle until they have caramelized on the bottom, about 2 minutes. When the bottoms are caramelized, toss them once and season with salt and pepper, to taste. Add the dill, oregano, crushed red pepper and pepper. Stir in the thawed spinach and artichokes and gently stir everything to combine. Cook another 2-3 minutes until heated through.

3. Add half of the pasta, the cubes of fontina and a drizzle of olive oil, toss well, adding in more pasta if desired. Create small wells for the eggs and carefully

crack the eggs into the wells. Sprinkle the eggs with salt and pepper and then add the remaining shredded cheese. Drizzle the cream over the eggs. Place the whole skillet in the oven and bake until the whites are just set but yolks are still runny, about 15 to 18 minutes. If you want to brown the cheese a bit more turn the broiler on for 30 seconds, but the eggs will probably not be runny anymore. Remove from the oven and add the crispy bacon. Garnish with chopped parsley. EAT!

Prep Time: 15 Minutes

Cook Time: 50 Minutes

Servings 12

Ingredients

Preferment:

- 1 cup bread flour
- 1/2 cup warm water
- 1/4 teaspoon active dry or instant yeast

Final Dough:

- 2 teaspoons active dry yeast
- 3 tablespoons honey plus more for drizzling
- 1 1/2 cups warm water divided
- 1 cup old fashions oats
- 3 tablespoons ground flax
- 1 1/2 cups white whole wheat flour
- 1 1/4 cups bread flour plus more for kneading
- 1 teaspoon salt
- 1 egg beaten

- 1 cup mixed pumpkin seeds sunflower seeds, black and or white sesame seeds and flax seeds)

Instructions

1. The night before baking the bread make the preferment. In the bowl of your stand mixer, mix together the flour, water and yeast until a smooth paste forms. Cover the bowl and allow the preferment to ripen at room temperature overnight. The preferment will double in size and become bubbly on top as it sits.

2. The next day measure out 1/4 cup warm water in a glass measuring cup or bowl. Add the yeast and honey. Mix to combine and then allow the mixture to sit, undisturbed for 5 minutes or until the mixture is foamy on top and smells like bread. During the same time add the remaining 1 1/4 cups warm water to a bowl. Add the oats and ground flax. Allow this mixture to sit 5 minutes.

3. After 5 minutes add both the yeast mixture and oats mixture to the bowl with the preferment from the night before. Add the whole wheat flour, bread flour and salt. Using the dough hook, mix the dough on

medium speed for 4-6 minutes. If the dough seems extremely sticky, add 1-2 tablespoons flour. Now add in 3-4 tablespoons of the mixed seeds. mix until combined.

4. Remove the dough from the bowl and knead with your hands on a floured surface for a minute or two.

5. Grease the bowl you mixed the dough in and place the dough back in the bowl. Cover with plastic wrap and place in a warm area for 1 1/2 to 2 hours or until the dough has doubled in size.

6. Once the dough has doubled in size, preheat to the oven 450 degrees F. Place a 5-quart, or larger, cast iron dutch oven with a tight fitting lid in the center of the rack. You may also use a baking stone, but I have found the the dutch oven with a lid works the best.

7. Punch the dough down with your fist and then scoop it out onto a floured work surface. Knead the dough a few times with your hands and then form the dough into rough oval or circle shape (if needed, you can divided the dough in half and make two loafs). Place the dough on a parchment lined baking sheet and cover with a damp kitchen towel. Allow the dough to rise 20-30 minutes.

8. After 20-30 minutes, brush the dough with the beaten egg and then sprinkle with the remaining mixed seeds. Using a sharp knife, gently make a small slit down the center of the loaf. Drizzle the the seeds with 1-2 teaspoons honey.

9. When the dough is ready to bake, carefully remove the hot dutch oven from the oven using oven mitts and remove the lid. Very carefully, pick the dough up by the parchment paper and lift into the hot dutch oven. Using oven mitts, place the hot lid back on the pot and return to the oven. Bake for 20 minutes, then reduce the heat to 375 degrees F. Using oven mitts, remove the hot lid and continue baking until the bread is a deep, golden brown, about 15-20 minutes more. Remove from the oven. Using a thin handle of a spatula, carefully lift the bread out of the pot and place it on a rack to cool completely, about 2 hours. Don't slice into the bread right out of the oven, the bread continues to cook as it cools.

Prep Time: 40 Minutes

Cook Time: 15 Minutes

Servings 16

Ingredients

- 1/4 cup warm water
- 1 tablespoon honey
- 2 1/4 teaspoons active dry yeast
- 1 1/2 cups apple cider, warm
- 1 stick (1/2 cup) salted butter, melted
- 4 1/2 cups all-purpose flour

Filling:

- 1/2 cup granulated sugar
- 4 teaspoons ground cinnamon
- 6 tablespoons salted butter, at room temperature
- 3/4 cup apple butter
- 1/2 cup brown sugar
- 1 tablespoon all-purpose flour

Instructions

1. Combine the water, honey, and yeast in the bowl of a stand mixer. Let sit for 5 minutes, until bubbly on top.

2. Add the apple cider, butter, and flour. Mix on medium speed until the dough is smooth and begins to pull away from the sides of the bowl, about 3 to 4 minutes. If the dough is too wet or too dry, add additional flour or water, 1 tablespoon at a time. Cover the bowl and place in a warm spot until the dough doubles in size, about 1-2 hours.

3. Meanwhile, mix the sugar and 2 teaspoons cinnamon in a bowl.

4. Preheat the oven to 425° F. Line 2 baking sheets with parchment.

5. On a floured surface, roll the dough out into a rectangle about 1/4 inch thick (about 16×14 inches), adding flour as needed. Spread the dough with 4 tablespoons butter, then the apple butter. Sprinkle with cinnamon sugar. Fold the dough in half, pressing to adhere. Cut into 16 strips. Twist each strip into a loose knot, it doesn't need to be perfect.

6. Melt 2 tablespoons butter. Add the brown sugar, flour, and 2 teaspoons cinnamon. Spoon clumps of the brown sugar mix over the knots (see above photo).

7. Bake for 15 to 18 minutes or until pretzels are golden
   brown. Enjoy warm or at room temp, warm is best

Prep Time: 15 Minutes

Cook Time: 45 Minutes

Servings 2

Ingredients

- 2 tablespoons extra virgin olive oil
- 2 heirloom tomatoes, sliced
- 4-6 cloves garlic, left in skin and smashed
- Salt and black pepper
- Red pepper flakes
- 1/4 cup basil pesto
- 4 slices sourdough bread
- 2 tablespoons fig preserves (optional)
- 1 1/2 cups shredded mozzarella
- 1/4 cup grated parmesan
- 1 cup fresh basil leaves
- 4 tablespoons salted butter, at room temperature

Instructions

1. Preheat oven to 425° F.

2. Arrange the tomato slices on a parchment-lined baking sheet. Scatter the smashed garlic cloves around the tomatoes. Drizzle everything with olive oil and season with salt pepper, and chili flakes. Bake 20-25 minutes, until tomatoes are deeply roasted.

3. Remove the garlic from the pan and pop the cloves out of the skin. Mash the cloves with a fork into a paste. Mix the roasted garlic with the basil pesto.

4. Brush the outside of each slice of bread with butter. On the inside of half of the slices of bread, spread with fig preserves. Evenly layer the cheeses, the tomatoes, pesto, and the remaining cheese. Add the top piece of bread.

5. Melt 1-2 tablespoons butter in a large skillet over medium heat. Place the sandwiches in the skillet and cook until golden on each side, about 3-5 minutes per side. EAT and ENJOY!

Prep Time: 20 Minutes

Cook Time: 15 Minutes

Servings 4

Ingredients

Strawberry Jam:

- 6 cups fresh sliced strawberries
- 1/3-1/2 cup maple syrup
- 2 teaspoons lemon juice
- 1 teaspoon vanilla bean powder (or 2 tsp vanilla extract)

Dutch Baby:

- 4 tablespoons salted butter, plus more for serving
- 4 large eggs, at room temperature
- 2/3 cups whole milk, at room temperature
- 2/3 cup all-purpose flour
- 1/2 teaspoon salt
- 2 teaspoons vanilla extract

Instructions

1. Preheat the oven to 450° F.

2. To make the jam. Add the strawberries, maple syrup, lemon juice, and vanilla to a medium-size pot set over high heat. Bring the mixture to a boil, once boiling, use a spoon to break down and mash the berries. Continue to cook for 5-8 minutes or until the jam has reduced and thickened by 1/3. Keep warm.

3. Meanwhile, bake the Dutch baby. Using an electric mixer, whisk together the eggs, milk, flour, salt, vanilla, and 2 tablespoons melted butter until the batter is smooth, about 1 minute. Make sure no large clumps of flour remain.

4. Melt the butter in a 10-12 inch cast iron skillet set over medium heat. Allow the butter to brown until it smells toasted and is a deep golden color, about 3-4 minutes. Pour the batter into the hot skillet. Place the skillet in the center of the oven and bake for 15 minutes or until the pancake is fully puffed and browned on top. DO NOT open the oven during the first 15 minutes of cooking or you might deflate your Dutch baby.

5. As soon as the Dutch baby comes out of the oven, top it with pats of butter, then warm jam. Cover the

surface with jam! Add whipped cream if you'd like,
Enjoy!

Prep Time: 15 Minutes

Cook Time: 40 Minutes

Servings 6

Ingredients

- 2 tablespoons + 3 teaspoons salted butter
- 1 1/2 cups whole milk, at room temperature
- 3 large eggs, at room temperature
- 1 1/2 cups all purpose flour
- 1/4 cup grated cheddar cheese
- 1 jalapeño, seeded and finely chopped
- 1 teaspoon salt
- 1/2 teaspoon onion powder
- 1/2 teaspoon garlic powder
- 4 tablespoons salted butter, at room temperature
- 3 tablespoons honey

Instructions

1. Heat 2 tablespoons butter in a small skillet over medium heat and cook the butter until it begins to bubble, then brown, 3-4 minutes.

2. Position a rack in the lower third of the oven. Preheat the oven to 450 degrees. Place 1/2 teaspoon of butter in each cup of a 6 cup standard popover pan. Alternately, you can use a 12-cup muffin pan and make 10 mini popovers. Place the pan on a baking sheet and then into the oven to melt the butter, 3-5 minutes.

3. In medium bowl, vigorously whisk together the milk and eggs until frothy, about 1 minute. Add the browned butter, flour, salt, onion powder and garlic powder. Whisk in the cheddar and jalapeño. It's OK if there are small lumps.

4. Remove the popover pan from the oven and swirl the butter around the cups to grease the pan. Evenly divide the batter between the popover cups, filling them about 3/4 of the way full. Bake for 20 minutes. Lower the oven temperature to 350 degrees. Bake another 10-20 minutes, until deeply golden.

5. Meanwhile, make the honey butter. In a small bowl, combine the butter, honey, and a pinch of flaky sea

salt. Serve the popovers warm with honey butter and flaky salt.

Prep Time: 5 Minutes

Cook Time: 10 Minutes

Servings 2

Ingredients

Chili Butter:

- 1 tablespoons extra virgin olive oil
- 2 tablespoons salted butter
- 1 clove garlic, chopped
- 1-2 teaspoon chili flakes (or Aleppo pepper)
- 1/2 teaspoon paprika

Eggs:

- 4 large eggs
- 1/2 cup finely shredded cheddar cheese
- Sea salt and black pepper
- Pieces sourdough or whole grain bread, toasted
- 1 small avocado, lightly mashed
- fresh herbs

Instructions

1. In a saucepan, melt together the olive oil, butter, garlic, chili flakes, and paprika. Let the butter bubble up and begin to brown, then remove from heat.
2. Place the eggs in a medium pot and cover with water by 1 inch. Bring to a boil over high heat, cover, and remove from the heat. Let sit 5 minutes for a softer yolk and 10 for hard boiled.
3. Drain the eggs, peel and slice into quarters. Add to a bowl with the cheese and season with salt. Use a fork to lightly mash the eggs and cheese together.
4. Spread the avocado on toast. Spoon over the eggs, then drizzle with chili butter. Dad didn't do this, but I love to top with herbs.

11. Tomato Peach Crostini with Hot Bacon Dressing

Prep Time: 15 Minutes

Cook Time: 15 Minutes

Servings 8

Ingredients

Dressing:

- 6 thick-cut slices of bacon, chopped
- 1/4 cup extra virgin olive oil
- 2 tablespoons champagne or white balsamic vinegar
- 1 tablespoon fig preserves or honey
- 1/4 cup fresh basil, chopped
- chili flakes
- Salt and black pepper

Crostini:

- 1/4 cup extra virgin olive oil
- 2 cloves garlic, chopped
- 1 sourdough or french baguette, sliced
- 1 log goat cheese, at room temperature

- 2 peaches, chopped or sliced
- 1 cup cherry tomatoes, halved

Instructions

1. To make the dressing. Combine all ingredients except the bacon in a glass jar and whisk until smooth.
2. Cook the bacon in a large skillet over medium heat until crisp. Drain onto a paper towel. Stir the bacon into the dressing.
3. Preheat your grill to high heat or preheat your oven to 400° F.
4. To make the crostini. Mix the olive oil, garlic, and a pinch of salt. Place the bread on a baking sheet and rub/drizzle with the garlic oil. Place the bread on the grill and grill both sides for 2-3 minutes per side or until lightly toasted. Remove from the grill.
5. Toss the peaches and tomatoes with a few tablespoons of dressing. Spread the goat cheese over the warm bread. Top with the dressing, peaches/tomatoes, and fresh basil. Drizzle over the remaining dressing.

Prep Time: 25 Minutes

Cook Time: 15 Minutes

Servings 4

Ingredients

Avocado Ranch:

- 1 small avocado, pitted and peeled
- 1/2 cup sour cream or plain Greek yogurt
- 1/4 cup pickled jalapeños
- 2 teaspoons lemon juice
- 3 tablespoons chopped fresh chives
- 2 tablespoons chopped fresh dill
- 1 teaspoon onion powder
- 1 teaspoon garlic powder
- Salt and black pepper

Wraps:

- 4 large tortillas
- gluten free tortillas (optional)
- 3 cups shredded lettuce
- 1 cup cooked quinoa

- 1-2 tablespoons fajita seasoning
- 1/2 cup shredded cheddar or pepper jack
- 1 cup cooked black beans
- 1 cup grilled or roasted corn
- 1 roasted/grilled bell pepper, sliced
- 1/2 cups grilled chicken, cubed or shredded
- 1 cup fresh cilantro, chopped

Instructions

1. To make the dressing. Combine all ingredients in a food processor or blender with 1/3 cup water. Blend until creamy, adding more water as needed to thin. Taste and adjust the salt and pepper.

2. To make the wraps. In a large salad bowl, combine the lettuce, quinoa, fajita seasoning, cheese, black beans, peppers, corn, and cilantro. Toss with 1/2 of the dressing.

3. Place one tortilla at a time in the microwave for 20 seconds. Spread on a layer of ranch then add the salad and chicken. Drizzle over more ranch and if you're feeling it, more fajita seasoning. Fold the tortilla over the ingredients. Fold sides and ends of tortillas over

filling and roll forward. Repeat with remaining ingredients.

4. Serve room temp or place in a skillet with olive oil to warm. Enjoy with extra dressing!

Prep Time: 30 Minutes

Cook Time: 20 Minutes

Servings 6

Ingredients

- 1 egg, beaten
- 1 pound boneless chicken tenders
- 1 cup finely crushed salted pretzel twists
- 1 tablespoon dried chives
- 1 tablespoon dried parsley
- 1 tablespoon dried dill
- 1/2 teaspoon garlic powder
- 1/2 teaspoon onion powder
- extra virgin olive oil
- 1/2 cup buffalo sauce
- 1 cup torn ciabatta bread
- 6 cups mixed greens
- 1 cup chopped celery
- 1/2 cup shaved parmesan
- 1-2 avocados, diced
- 4 ounces crumbled blue cheese

- 4 slices cooked thick cut bacon, crumbled

Caesar Dressing:

- 1/2 cup mayo
- 3 tablespoons extra virgin olive oil
- 3 tablespoons lemon juice
- 2 teaspoons dijon mustard
- 2 teaspoons Worcestershire sauce
- 1-2 cloves garlic, grated
- Salt and black pepper
- 1/3 cup grated parmesan

Instructions

1. Preheat the oven to 425° F. Line a baking sheet with parchment.
2. In a bowl, whisk the eggs. Add the chicken and toss to coat. Combine the pretzels, chives, parsley, dill, garlic powder, onion powder, and a pinch of pepper in a bowl.
3. Dredge the chicken through the crumbs, pressing to adhere. Place on the prepared baking sheet. Drizzle the chicken with olive oil. Bake for 15-20 minutes or until the chicken is cooked through.

4. Toss the hot chicken in buffalo sauce.

5. To make the salad. Combine the greens, breadcrumbs, blue cheese (or use cheddar or parmesan), avocados, and bacon in a salad bowl.

6. To make the dressing. Combine all ingredients in a glass jar and whisk until smooth. Taste and adjust the salt and pepper. Toss the salad with the dressing, saving some for serving.

7. Toss the chicken in with the salad. Add a little more of the dressing and extra buffalo sauce. Enjoy!

Prep Time: 20 Minutes

Cook Time: 10 Minutes

Servings 6

Ingredients

Dressing:

- 6 thick-cut slices of bacon, chopped
- 1/4 cup extra virgin olive oil
- 1 shallot, thinly sliced
- 1-2 cloves garlic, grated
- 3 tablespoons apple cider vinegar
- 1 tablespoon fig preserves
- 1 tablespoon fresh thyme leaves
- chili flakes
- salt and pepper

Salad:

- 1 cup torn ciabatta bread
- 1 clove garlic, grated
- 6 cups mixed salad greens
- 2 cups grilled chicken, cubed or shredded

- 1-2 roasted/grilled bell peppers, sliced
- 3 ears grilled corn, kernels removed from the cob
- 2 cups cherry tomatoes, halved
- 1 avocado, sliced
- 1/2 cup crumbled blue cheese or feta cheese

Instructions

1. To make the dressing. Combine all ingredients except the bacon in a glass jar and whisk until smooth.
2. Cook the bacon in a large skillet over medium heat until crisp. Drain onto a paper towel. Stir the bacon into the dressing.
3. To make the croutons. Heat the same skillet used to cook the bacon over medium heat. Add the bread and toss in the bacon grease. If needed add 1-2 tablespoons olive oil. Cook until toasted, 5 minutes, stirring occasionally. Add the garlic, then remove from the heat and season with salt.
4. To assemble the salad. In a large salad bowl, combine the greens, chicken, peppers, corn, tomatoes, avocado, cheese, and croutons. Toss well with the dressing. Enjoy!

Prep Time: 30 Minutes

Cook Time: 15 Minutes

Servings 6

Ingredients

Dressing:

- 1/3 cup extra virgin olive oil
- 1 tablespoon honey
- 3 tablespoons dijon mustard
- 3 tablespoons lemon juice
- 2 tablespoons apple cider vinegar
- 1/2 cup mixed chopped herbs (basil, parsley, dill)
- 1 shallot, chopped
- 2 cloves garlic, grated
- salt, black pepper, and chili flakes

Sandwich:

- 3/4 pound boneless skinless chicken tenders
- 1 loaf ciabatta bread halved lengthwise

- sourdough sandwich bread
- 1 avocado, mashed
- 1/4 cup oil packed sun-dried tomatoes, drained and sliced
- 2 tablespoons chopped pepperoncini
- 1 cup baby arugula
- 1/2 cup shaved parmesan

Tahini Ranch:

- 1/4 cup tahini
- 2 tablespoons lemon juice
- 1 teaspoon dijon mustard
- 2 teaspoons dried chives
- 2 teaspoons dried parsley
- 1 teaspoon dried dill
- 1/2 teaspoon garlic powder
- 1/2 teaspoon onion powder
- 1/4– 1/2 teaspoon cayenne pepper, to taste

Instructions

1. To make the dressing. Combine all ingredients in a glass jar and whisk until smooth. Taste and adjust the salt and pepper.

2. In a large bowl, toss the chicken with 1/2 of the dressing. Let sit 10 minutes. Set your grill, grill pan, or skillet to medium-high heat. Grill the chicken until lightly charred and cooked through, turning halfway through cooking, about 10 to 12 minutes.

3. To make the tahini ranch, combine everything in a bowl, whisking in 1/4 to 1/2 cup water to thin the dressing. Taste and season with salt and pepper.

4. Rub each half of the bread with olive oil. Grill the bread, cut side down, for 3-5 minutes or until light grill marks appear.

5. Working with the bottom piece of bread, spread over some of the tahini ranch, then layer on the avocado, sun-dried tomatoes, and pepperoncini. Add the chicken, then drizzle the remaining dressing over the chicken. Add the arugula and cheese. Drizzle with the tahini ranch. Add the top half of the ciabatta and gently push down on the sandwich. Cut into 4-6 sandwiches. Enjoy with the remaining tahini ranch on the side.

Prep Time: 25 Minutes

Cook Time: 10 Minutes

Servings 6

Ingredients

Greek Dressing:

- 1/4 cup extra virgin olive oil
- 3 tablespoons lemon juice
- 3 tablespoons red wine vinegar
- 2 tablespoons tahini or mayo
- 2 teaspoons dijon mustard
- 2 teaspoons honey
- salt and black pepper

Salad:

- 2 shallots, thinly sliced
- 1/2 cup mixed fresh herbs (basil, oregano, dill)
- 2 tablespoons pine nuts
- chili flakes
- 1/4 cup extra virgin olive oil
- 1 pound short cut pasta

- 3/4 cup mixed Greek olives, pitted
- 2 bell peppers, chopped
- 1 cup chopped cucumber
- 1 cup cherry tomatoes, halved
- 1 cup canned chickpeas, drained
- 1/4 cup sliced pepperoncini
- 8 ounces feta cheese, crumbled

Instructions

1. To make the dressing. Combine all ingredients in a glass jar and whisk until smooth. Taste and adjust the salt and pepper.
2. To make the salad. Combine the shallots, pine nuts, herbs, and chili flakes in a large bowl. Heat the olive oil in a small skillet over medium heat until it begins to sizzle. Pour the hot oil over the shallots.
3. Bring a large pot of salted water to a boil. Boil the pasta to al dente, according to package directions. Drain. Add the pasta to the bowl with the oil. Add the olives, peppers, tomatoes, chickpeas, and pepperoncini. Pour over the dressing and toss well. Add the feta.
4. Serve the salad warm or cold and enjoy!

Prep Time: 25 Minutes

Cook Time: 25 Minutes

Servings 6

Ingredients

- 2 sheets frozen puff pastry, thawed
- 1 egg, beaten
- 1 tablespoon sesame seeds
- black pepper
- 1 cup shredded gouda cheese
- 1 cup shredded fontina cheese
- 3 tablespoons chopped peppercinis
- 1/4 cup chopped fresh basil
- 2 tablespoons fresh thyme leaves
- 3 cloves garlic, chopped
- 1 tbsp lemon zest
- chili flakes
- 1 jar (14 ounce or two 7.5 oz jars) marinated artichokes, drained
- honey, for drizzling

Instructions

1. Preheat the oven to 425° F. Line a baking sheet with parchment paper.

2. Roll the puff pastry out a little to stretch it and then transfer to the prepared baking sheet. Brush the edges of the pastry with the beaten egg. Take the second sheet of pastry and cut 4 (1/2 inch) wide strips. Stick the strips around the edges of the larger sheet of pastry, pressing to adhere. Brush the edges of the big pastry sheet with the egg, then sprinkle with sesame seeds and black pepper. Prick the inside of the pastry all over with a fork (see above photos).

3. Working inside the borders, arrange the peppercinis , basil, thyme, garlic, lemon zest, and chili flakes on the pastry. Then evenly sprinkle the cheeses over top. Add the artichokes and lightly drizzle over a squeeze of honey. Chill in the freezer for 10 minutes.

4. Bake for 25-30 minutes or until the pastry is golden and the cheese is melted.

18. Greek Chicken Tzatziki Bowls

Prep Time: 25 Minutes

Cook Time: 20 Minutes

Servings 6

Ingredients

- 1/3 cup full-fat plain Greek yogurt
- 1/4 cup extra virgin olive oil
- 1 1/2 pounds boneless skinless chicken breasts or thighs, cubed
- 6 garlic cloves, chopped
- 2 shallots, chopped
- 1 tablespoon smoked paprika
- 1 tablespoon chopped fresh oregano
- chili flakes, Kosher salt, and black pepper
- 2 Persian cucumbers, chopped
- 1 avocado, diced
- 2 tablespoons lemon juice
- 1/4 cup fresh dill, chopped
- 6 ounces crumbled feta cheese
- 1-2 cups Tzakiki sauce

- lettuce, peperoncini, onion, tomatoes, and pitas, for serving

Ginger Tahini:

- 1/2 cup tahini
- 2 teaspoons grated ginger
- 1 clove garlic, grated
- 2 teaspoons tamari
- 1 tablespoon lemon juice
- 2 teaspoons honey

Instructions

1. In a bowl, combine the yogurt, olive oil, cubed chicken, garlic, shallots, paprika, oregano, chili flakes, and a large pinch each of salt and pepper. Let marinate for 15 minutes at room temperature or up to overnight in the refrigerator.
2. Preheat the oven to 425° F. Arrange the chicken on a baking sheet. Bake 15 minutes, toss and bake another 5-10 minutes, or until cooked through. Switch the oven to broil. Broil 1-2 minutes, until the chicken chars on the edges.

3. Meanwhile, combine the cucumbers, avocado, lemon, dill, salt, and pepper.

4. To make the tahini. Combine all ingredients and 1/4 cup water in a blender and blend until smooth. If needed, add water to thin the sauce as desired. Season to taste with salt.

5. To assemble, add lettuce to a bowl. Top with chicken, cucumber/avocado, feta cheese, and any other desired toppings. Add a few dollops of Tzaziki sauce. Drizzle over the tahini.

Prep Time: 30 Minutes

Cook Time: 15 Minutes

Servings 6

Ingredients

Wontons:

- 3/4 pound ground chicken or pork
- 1 1/2 cups shredded cabbage
- 1 tablespoon fresh grated ginger
- 1 clove garlic, grated
- 4 green onions, chopped
- 1/4 cup tamari or soy sauce
- pinch of black pepper
- 24-26 square wonton wrappers

Chile Oil:

- 3/4 cup sesame oil
- 1 tablespoon fresh grated ginger
- 2 cloves garlic, grated
- 1 tablespoon chile sauce
- 1-3 tablespoons chili flakes, to taste

- 1 teaspoon paprika
- 3 tablespoons sesame seeds
- 1 teaspoon honey
- 3 tablespoons tamari or soy sauce
- 1 bunch asparagus, ends trimmed

Instructions

1. To make the wontons, combine all ingredients in a bowl except the wrappers.
2. To assemble, spoon 2 teaspoons of filling onto each wrapper. Brush water around the edges of the wrapper. Fold the edges of the wrapper up and around the filling and pinch to seal. Repeat with the remaining filling.
3. To make the chili oil. Combine the ginger, garlic, chile sauce, chili flakes, paprika, 2 tablespoons sesame seeds, and honey in a heat proof bowl. Heat the oil in a skillet over medium heat until it sizzles, 5 minutes. Pour the oil over the spices, stir to combine, then add 2 tablespoons tamari/soy sauce.
4. In the same skillet, cook the asparagus over medium heat until tender, 3-5 minutes. Turn the heat off and

add 1 tablespoon tamari/soy sauce and 1 tablespoon sesame seeds. Toss to combine.

5. Bring a large pot of salted water to a boil. Boil the wontons until they float, 3-4 minutes. Toss the warm wontons in the chili oil. If desired, spoon over some of the hot wonton cooking water to create a spicy broth. Serve the asparagus on the side.

Prep Time: 20 Minutes

Cook Time: 10 Minutes

Servings 4

Ingredients

- 2 strips thick cut bacon, chopped
- 2 cups sliced wild or cremini mushrooms
- 1 tablespoon chopped ginger
- 2 cloves garlic, chopped
- 2-4 tablespoons red curry paste
- 4 cups low sodium chicken broth
- 1/4 cup tamari or soy sauce
- 2 tablespoons rice vinegar
- 2 boneless, skinless chicken breasts
- 1 ounce dried porcini mushrooms
- 2 tablespoons toasted sesame oil
- 4 squares brown rice ramen noodles
- 3 cups fresh baby spinach
- soft boiled eggs, chili crisp sauce, shredded carrots, and green onions, for serving

Quick Honey Roasted Squash (Optional):

- 1 small acorn squash, cut into 6-8 wedges
- 1 tablespoon honey

Instructions

Instant Pot

1. Set Instant pot to sauté. Add the bacon and cook until crisp, about 5 minutes. Stir in the mushrooms, let cook 2 minutes. Add the ginger, garlic, and curry paste. Cook another minute, until fragrant.
2. Pour in the broth, 2 cups of water, the tamari, rice vinegar, chicken, dried porcini mushrooms, and sesame oil. If using, add the squash on top. Cover and cook on high pressure for 8 minutes.
3. Once done cooking, release the steam. Set the Instant pot to sauté. Remove the squash from the soup and place on a baking sheet. Set aside. Shred the chicken. Stir in the noodles and spinach. Let sit 5 minutes or until the noodles are soft.
4. To finish the squash, heat the broiler to high. Rub the squash with honey and season with salt, pepper, and chili flakes. Broil 2-3 minutes, until crisp.

5. To serve, ladle the soup into bowls and top with roasted squash and any other desired toppings. Enjoy!

Crockpot

1. Cook the bacon in a skillet oven set over medium heat until crisp, about 5 minutes. Transfer to the bowl of the crockpot. Stir in the mushrooms, ginger, garlic, and curry paste.
2. Pour in the broth, 2 cups of water, the tamari, rice vinegar, chicken, dried porcini mushrooms, and sesame oil. If using, add the squash on top. Cover and cook 4-6 hours on low or 2-3 hours high.
3. Remove the squash from the soup and place on a baking sheet. Set aside. Shred the chicken. Stir in the noodles and spinach. Let sit 5 minutes or until the noodles are soft.
4. Finish as directed about through step 4.

Stove

1. Cook the bacon in a large dutch oven set over medium heat until crisp, about 5 minutes. Stir in the mushrooms, let cook 2 minutes. Add the ginger, garlic, and curry paste. Cook another minute, until fragrant.

2. Pour in the broth, 2 cups of water, the tamari, rice vinegar, chicken, dried porcini mushrooms, and sesame oil. If using, add the squash on top. Cover and cook 15-20 minutes, until the chicken has cooked.

3. When tender, remove the squash from the soup and place on a baking sheet. Set aside. Shred the chicken. Stir in the noodles and spinach. Let sit 5 minutes or until the noodles are soft.

4. Finish as directed about through step 4.

21. Creamy Butternut Squash Butter Chicken

Prep Time: 20 Minutes

Cook Time: 25 Minutes

Servings 6

Ingredients

- 1 1/2 pounds boneless skinless chicken breasts/thighs, cut into bite-size chunks
- 1/4 cup plain Greek yogurt
- 2 teaspoons plus 1 tablespoon garam masala
- 1 teaspoons paprika
- 2 teaspoons cumin
- 1 teaspoon turmeric
- 1-2 teaspoons cayenne pepper, use to taste
- salt and black pepper
- 2 tablespoons extra virgin olive oil
- 4 tablespoons salted butter
- 1 large yellow onion, chopped
- 2 cups cubed butternut squash
- 6 cloves garlic, chopped

- 2 tablespoons fresh grated ginger
- 1-2 teaspoons chili flakes, use to taste
- 1 tablespoon tomato paste
- 1 (14 ounce) can full-fat coconut milk
- 1/2 cup fresh cilantro, roughly chopped

Instructions

1. in a bowl, toss together the chicken, yogurt, 2 teaspoons garam masala, 1 teaspoon cumin, 1/2 teaspoon paprika, 1/2 teaspoon turmeric, 1/2 – 1 teaspoon cayenne pepper, and 1 teaspoon salt. Let sit 5-10 minutes.
2. Heat the oil in a large skillet over medium-high heat. Add the chicken and sear on both sides until browned, about 2 minutes. Add 2 tablespoons of butter and toss to coat the chicken. Remove the chicken from the skillet to a plate.
3. To the skillet, add the onion and butternut squash, tossing with the butter in the skillet. Cook 5 minutes, until softened. Add 2 tablespoons butter, the garlic, ginger, 1 tablespoon garam masala, 1 teaspoon cumin, 1/2 teaspoon paprika, 1/2 teaspoon turmeric, 1/2 – 1 teaspoon cayenne pepper, paprika, and the chili

flakes. Season with salt and pepper. Cook until fragrant, about 5 minutes. Add the tomato paste and continue cooking another 3-4 minutes.

4. Reduce the heat to low. Add 1 cup water and the coconut milk. Stir to combine, bring the sauce to a simmer, cook 5 minutes or until the sauce thickens slightly. If the sauce seems too thick, thin with 1/2 to 1 cup additional coconut milk. Add the chicken and any juices in the pan and cook, stirring occasionally, until the sauce thickens slightly, about 10 minutes. Remove from the heat and stir in the cilantro. Season with salt and pepper.

5. Serve the chicken, squash, and sauce over bowls of rice with fresh naan. Enjoy!

Prep Time: 15 Minutes

Cook Time: 30 Minutes

Servings 6

Ingredients

- 2 tablespoons extra virgin olive oil
- 1 medium yellow onion, chopped
- 2 poblano peppers, seeded and chopped
- 4 cloves garlic, chopped
- 1 tablespoon dried parsley
- 1 tablespoon dried chives
- 2 teaspoons dried dill
- 1 teaspoon smoked paprika
- Salt
- black pepper
- 1 pound boneless skinless chicken breasts or thighs
- 4-6 cups low-sodium chicken broth
- 4 ounces cream cheese, at room temperature
- 1 can white beans, drained
- 3/4 cup buffalo sauce
- 1/2 cup salsa verde

- 1 cup shredded cheddar cheese
- 1/2 cup fresh cilantro, chopped
- avocado, cheddar cheese, and Greek yogurt, for serving

Instructions

Stove

1. Heat the olive oil in a large pot over medium heat. Add the onion and poblano peppers cook until fragrant, about 5 minutes. Stir in the garlic, parsley, chives, dill, paprika, and a pinch each of salt and pepper. Cook 5 minutes, until very fragrant. Add the chicken, then stir in 4 cups broth. Season with salt and pepper. Partially cover and simmer over medium-low heat for 20 minutes, until the chicken is cooked through.
2. Pull the chicken out and shred using 2 forks.
3. Stir in the cream cheese until smooth, slowly letting it melt into the broth. Add the shredded chicken, white beans, salsa verde, buffalo sauce, and cheddar cheese. Cook 5-10 minutes, until the cheese is melted. Remove from the heat and stir in the cilantro. If needed, thin with additional broth.

4. Ladle the chili into bowls. Top, as desired, with Greek yogurt/sour cream, cheese, avocado, cilantro, and green onions. Eat and enjoy!

Crockpot

1. In the bowl of your crockpot, combine the onion, poblano peppers, garlic, parsley, chives, dill, and paprika. Add the chicken, then stir in 4 cups broth and cream cheese. Season with salt and pepper.

2. Cover and cook on low for 6-7 hours or high for 4-5 hours.

3. Shred the chicken using two forks. Stir in the white beans, salsa verde, buffalo sauce, cheddar, and cilantro.

4. Ladle the chili into bowls. Top, as desired, with Greek yogurt/sour cream, cheese, avocado, cilantro, and green onions. Eat and enjoy!

Prep Time: 35 Minutes

Cook Time: 25 Minutes

Servings 6

Ingredients

Dumplings:

- 4 cups cubed butternut squash
- 2 tablespoons extra virgin olive oil
- 1 tablespoon spicy/regular curry powder
- 2 teaspoons honey
- 2 green onions chopped
- black pepper
- 24-26 round dumplings or wonton wrappers
- 1/4 cup sesame seeds

Ginger Broth:

- 2 tablespoons salted butter or olive oil
- 3-4 medium shallots, sliced
- 1 tablespoon chopped fresh ginger
- 2 cloves garlic, chopped
- 1/3 cup dry white wine

- 4 cups low sodium chicken/vegetable broth
- 1/3 cup tamari/soy sauce
- 1 cinnamon stick (or use 1/4 teaspoon cinnamon)
- chili crisp sauce, for serving

Instructions

1. Preheat the oven to 425° F. On a baking sheet, toss together the butternut squash, olive oil, and curry powder. Bake for 25-30 minutes, or until tender.
2. Add the squash, green onions, honey, and a pinch of pepper to a bowl. Mash together with a fork.
3. To assemble, spoon 1 tablespoon of filling onto each wrapper. Brush water around the edges of the wrapper. Fold the edges of the wrapper up and around the filling and pinch in the center to seal. Repeat with the remaining wrappers.
4. Place the sesame seeds in a shallow bowl. Brush the bottoms of the dumplings with water and then dredge them in the sesame seeds.
5. To make the broth. Melt together the butter and shallots in a large skillet over medium-high heat. Cook until softened, about 5 minutes. Add the wine, cooking until the wine cooks into the shallots, another

5 to 10 minutes, or until the shallots have caramelized. Add ginger and garlic and cook 1 minute. Add the broth, soy sauce, and cinnamon. Simmer over low heat.

6. Heat a few tablespoons of oil in a large skillet set over medium heat. Add the dumplings and cook until the bottoms are golden brown, 2-3 minutes. Carefully pour 1/4 cup of water into the skillet. Immediately cover. Turn the heat to medium-low and let the dumplings steam for 4-5 minutes. Remove the dumplings from the skillet to a plate.

7. Arrange the dumplings in shallow bowls. Ladle the steaming broth over top. Top with chili crisp sauce and green onions. Enjoy!

Prep Time: 15 Minutes

Cook Time: 15 Minutes

Servings 8

Ingredients

- 2 tablespoons extra virgin olive oil
- 2 yellow onions, thinly sliced
- Salt and black pepper
- 3/4 cup apple cider
- 1/2 pound pizza dough, homemade or store-bought
- 1 cup cooked shredded chicken
- 1/2 cup BBQ sauce
- 2 tablespoons chopped fresh chives
- 1/2 cup fresh cilantro or parsley, chopped
- 1/4 cup ranch dressing (homemade sauce)
- 1 cup shredded whole milk mozzarella
- 1 cup shredded gouda or cheddar cheese
- 1/2 cup grated parmesan
- fresh herbs

Instructions

1. Position the oven rack in the upper 1/3 portion of your oven. Preheat the oven to 500° F.
2. Place the pizza dough on a lightly oiled quarter sheet pan. Gently press the dough until it covers most of the sheet pan. Cover and let sit while you prep the pizza.
3. In a large skillet set over medium-high heat combine the olive oil, onions, and a pinch of salt. Cook 5 minutes, until softened. Add half the apple cider and continue cooking another 5 minutes, until the cider has mostly evaporated. Add the remaining cider and cook another 5 minutes or until the onions are golden and caramelized. Remove from the heat.
4. In a bowl, combine the chicken, 1/3 cup BBQ sauce, chives, and cilantro/parsley.
5. To assemble. Grab the dough and spread on the ranch, you may not need it all. Add a drizzle of BBQ sauce if you'd like, then layer on the onions, chicken, and cheeses. Sprinkle with cilantro. Slide into the preheated oven and bake for 10 minutes, rotate the pizza, and bake another 3-5 minutes or until the crust is golden and the cheese has melted. Top the pizza with fresh herbs, additional BBQ sauce, and/or ranch. ENJOY!

Prep Time: 15 Minutes

Cook Time: 3hrs 15 Minutes

Servings 6

Ingredients

- 2 pounds boneless chicken breasts
- 1 tablespoon extra virgin olive oil
- 1 tablespoon dijon mustard
- 1 tablespoon fresh thyme leaves
- 2 tablespoons fresh chopped sage
- 1 head garlic, cloves peeled and left whole
- Salt and black pepper
- 3/4 cup dry white wine, such as Pinot Grigio or Sauvignon Blanc
- 2 tablespoons lemon juice
- 2 tablespoons salted butter
- 1 pound potato or cauliflower gnocchi
- 1 1/2 cups shredded brussels sprouts
- 1/3 cup heavy cream or canned full fat coconut milk
- 1/3 cup freshly grated parmesan cheese
- fresh basil for serving

Instructions

Crockpot

1. In the bowl of your slow cooker, rub the chicken with the olive oil, mustard, sage, thyme, salt, and pepper. Add the garlic cloves. Pour over the wine and lemon juice. Add the parmesan rind, if using. Cover and cook on low for 3-4 hours or on high for 1-2 hours.
2. Preheat the broiler to high. Remove the chicken from the slow cooker place it on a baking sheet.
3. Crank the heat on the slow cooker to high. Stir in the gnocchi, brussels sprouts, and 1/2 cup water. Cover and cook 15 minutes, or until the gnocchi soft. Stir in the cream and parmesan.
4. Place the butter on the chicken, then broil 1-3 minutes, until crisp. Serve the chicken over the gnocchi with fresh basil on top. Enjoy!

Instant Pot

1. Set the instant pot to sauté. Rub the chicken with the olive oil, mustard, sage, thyme, garlic, salt, and pepper. Add the chicken to the instant pot and sear until golden brown on both sides, about 3 minutes per side. Add the garlic cloves. Pour over the wine and lemon juice. Add the parmesan rind, if using, and

butter. Cover and cook on high pressure for 6 minutes.

2. Once done cooking, release the steam. Set the Instant pot to sauté. Stir in the gnocchi, brussels sprouts, and 1/2 cup water. Cook 6-8 minutes, until soft. Stir in the cream and parmesan.

3. Serve the chicken over the gnocchi with fresh basil on top. Enjoy!

Stove-Top

1. Heat a large dutch oven over medium-high heat. Rub the chicken with the olive oil, mustard sage, thyme, garlic, salt, and pepper. Add the chicken to the pot and sear until golden brown on both sides, about 3 minutes per side. Reduce the heat to medium. Pour in the wine and lemon juice. Add the butter. Cover and cook 10 minutes.

2. Stir in the gnocchi, brussels sprouts, and 1/2 cup water. Cook, stirring often, another 6-8 minutes, or until soft. Stir in the cream and parmesan.

3. Serve the chicken over the gnocchi with fresh basil on top. Enjoy!

Prep Time: 15 Minutes

Cook Time: 30 Minutes

Servings 6

Ingredients

- 1 1/2 pounds thin cut chicken breasts
- Salt and black pepper
- 1/4 cup all-purpose or gluten free flour
- 2 tablespoons extra virgin olive oil
- 3 ounces prosciutto, torn
- 2 shallots, chopped
- 4 cloves garlic, chopped
- 2 tablespoons Italian seasoning
- 1/2 cup oil-packed sun-dried tomatoes, chopped
- red pepper flakes
- 3 cups low sodium chicken broth
- 1 cup peeled and chopped raw potatoes
- 3/4 cup heavy cream or canned coconut milk
- 1 tablespoon dijon mustard
- 3 tablespoons lemon juice
- 1/2 cup grated parmesan cheese

- 1 bunch Tuscan kale, roughly chopped
- fresh basil

Instructions

1. Season the chicken with salt and pepper. Sprinkle with Italian seasoning. Place the flour in a shallow bowl and dredge the chicken through the flour, pressing to adhere.
2. Heat 1 tablespoon olive oil in a large skillet set over medium-high heat. Add the prosciutto and cook until crispy all over, about 5 minutes. Remove from the skillet.
3. In the same skillet, add 1 tablespoon olive oil and the chicken and sear on both sides until golden, about 3-5 minutes per side. Remove from the skillet.
4. Add the shallots and garlic and cook until fragrant, 2 minutes. Stir in the sun-dried tomatoes, Italian seasoning, and a pinch each of red pepper flakes, salt, and pepper. Cook 2 minutes. Pour in the broth. Add the potatoes and chicken. Partially cover and cook over medium heat until the potatoes are fork tender, 10-15 minutes.

5. Remove the lid. Pour in the cream. Add the dijon, lemon juice, parmesan, and Tuscan kale. Cook until the kale is wilted, 5 minutes.

6. Serve the chicken and sauce with crispy prosciutto and fresh basil.

Prep Time: 15 Minutes

Cook Time: 15 Minutes

Servings 6

Ingredients

- 2 tablespoons salted butter
- 2 tablespoons extra virgin olive oil
- 3 cloves garlic, chopped
- 1 tablespoon chopped fresh oregano
- chili flakes
- 1/3 cup tomato paste
- 2 cups Anellini or other small pasta
- salt and black pepper
- 1 teaspoon onion powder
- 1/2 teaspoon paprika
- 1 cup grated parmesan cheese
- 1/2 cup grated pecorino cheese
- 1/2 cup fresh basil

Instructions

1. Melt together the butter, olive oil, garlic, oregano, and chili flakes in a large pot over medium heat. Cook until the butter turns golden, about 5 minutes.

2. Reduce the heat to low, stir in the tomato paste. Cook 1-2 minutes, then pour over 3 cups of water. Bring to a boil over high heat. Add the pasta, onion powder, paprika, and season with salt and pepper. Cook, stirring often, until the pasta is al dente, about 12 minutes.

3. Stir in the parmesan, pecorino, and basil until the cheese is melted.

4. Serve immediately topped with fresh basil. Eat!

Prep Time: 25 Minutes

Cook Time: 15 Minutes

Servings 4

Ingredients

- 4 salmon filets, cut into bite-size chunks
- 1 egg white
- 1/2 cup sesame seeds
- olive oil, for drizzling
- 1/4 cup tamari or soy sauce
- 3 tablespoons honey
- 1-2 tablespoons chili sauce
- 2 tablespoon toasted sesame oil
- 1 tablespoon grated fresh ginger
- 3-4 cups cooked rice

Herb Salad:

- 2 avocados, diced
- 2 small cucumbers, chopped
- 1/2 cup fresh basil, chopped
- 1/2 cup fresh cilantro, chopped

- 1/2 cup cherry tomatoes, halved
- 2 tablespoons lemon or lime juice
- Salt

Spicy Mayo:

- 1/2 cup mayo
- 1-2 tablespoons sriracha
- 2 teaspoons toasted sesame oil

Instructions

1. Preheat the oven to 450° F. Grease a baking sheet with olive oil.
2. Place the sesame seeds in a shallow bowl. Add the egg white to a separate bowl. Toss each piece of salmon through the egg, then coat in seeds. Place on the prepared baking sheet in a single layer.
3. Drizzle the salmon with olive oil. Bake 10-15 minutes or until the salmon is cooked to your liking.
4. In a small bowl, whisk together the tamari, honey, chili sauce, toasted sesame oil, and ginger. Set the sauce aside for serving.
5. To make the salad. Combine all ingredients in a bowl. Season with salt.

6. For the spicy mayo, combine all ingredients in a bowl.

7. Spoon the salmon over the bowls of rice. Top with the herb salad and drizzle the soy ginger sauce over everything. Add a dollop of spicy mayo. Enjoy!

Prep Time: 15 Minutes

Cook Time: 15 Minutes

Servings 6

Ingredients

- 2 tablespoons sesame oil
- 2 pounds boneless skinless chicken breast, cubed
- 2 tablespoons regular or spicy curry powder
- 3-4 tablespoons red curry paste
- 1 tablespoon tomato paste
- 2 tablespoons salted butter
- 2 garlic, chopped
- 1 tablespoon chopped fresh ginger
- 2 cups chopped broccoli florets
- 2 1/2 cups canned coconut milk
- 1/2 cup fresh chopped cilantro

Instructions

1. In a large skillet, combine the oil, chicken, curry powder, and a pinch of salt. Set over medium-high

heat, then cook 3 minutes. Add the curry paste, tomato paste, butter, garlic, and ginger. Cook another 2 minutes.

2. Add the broccoli, then pour in the coconut milk. Season with salt. Cook 5-10 minutes until the chicken is cooked through and the sauce has thickened.

3. Stir in the cilantro. Serve the chicken and sauce over rice and with mango topping on the side (recipe below).

Sesame Mango Topping:

1. In a bowl, mix 1 diced mango, 1 cup chopped cilantro, 2 tablespoons toasted sesame seeds, 2 tablespoons lemon juice, and a pinch of chili flakes. Serve with the chicken.

Prep Time: 15 Minutes

Cook Time: 15 Minutes

Servings 4

Ingredients

Salad:

- 1 cup shredded carrots
- 1 bell pepper, sliced
- 1/2 cup cherry tomatoes, halved
- 2 green onions, chopped
- 2 tablespoons toasted sesame oil
- 2 tablespoons lime juice
- 1 tablespoon rice vinegar
- 1 tablespoon fish sauce or tamari
- 2 teaspoons honey

Beef:

- 1 pound lean ground beef (or chicken or pork)
- 4 cloves garlic, chopped
- 1 tablespoon fresh grated ginger
- black pepper

- 1/3 cup tamari or soy sauce
- 1/3 cup sweet Thai chili sauce (homemade in notes)
- 2 cups Thai or sweet Italian basil, chopped
- sesame seeds and peanuts, for serving

Instructions

1. To make the salad. Combine all ingredients in a bowl. Toss well and set aside.
2. To make the beef. In a large skillet, cook the beef with black pepper over medium heat, breaking up the meat as it cooks until browned, about 5 minutes. Add the garlic and ginger and cook another minute. Add the tamari, sweet Thai chili sauce, and 1 cup of fresh basil. Bring the mixture to a simmer and cook until the sauce coats the beef, 3-5 minutes. Remove from the heat and stir in the remaining basil.
3. Divide the rice and beef between bowls. Add the salad to the bowl. Top with peanuts, sesame seeds, and fresh basil. Enjoy!

Lemongrass Rice:

1. Add 1 can coconut milk and 1/3 water to a medium-sized pot. Bring to a low boil. Add in 1 1/2 cups

jasmine rice and 1 tablespoon lemongrass paste. Stir to combine. Place the lid on the pot and turn the heat down to the lowest setting possible. Allow the rice to cook ten minutes on low and then turn the heat off completely. Let the rice sit on the stove, covered, for another 15-20 minutes (don't take any peeks inside!).

2. After 15-20 minutes remove the lid and fluff the rice with a fork. Note that rice can cook differently for everyone, this is just what works for me.

www.ingramcontent.com/pod-product-compliance
Lightning Source LLC
Chambersburg PA
CBHW061511250726
48657CB00005B/1804